Using Food as a Psychological Weapon

Knowing More about Comfort Foods and Sugar Addiction

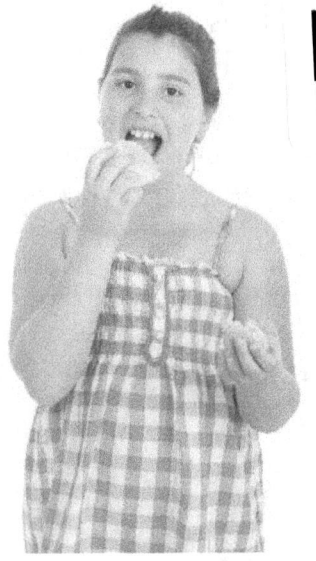

Dueep Jyot Singh

Healthy Learning Series

Mendon Cottage Books

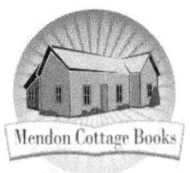

JD-Biz Publishing

Download Free Books!

http://MendonCottageBooks.com

Disclaimer

The information is this book is provided for informational purposes only. The information is believed to be accurate as presented based on research by the author.

The author or publisher is not responsible for the use or safety of any procedure or treatment mentioned in this book. The author or publisher is not responsible for errors or omissions that may exist.

Our books are available at

1. Amazon.com
2. Barnes and Noble
3. Itunes
4. Kobo
5. Smashwords
6. Google Play Books

Download Free Books!

http://MendonCottageBooks.com

Table of Contents

Introduction 4

Psychological Reasons for Unhealthy Eating Habits 6

Comfort Foods 8

Collecting All Those Muffins 13

Food As a Symbol of Love and Affection 15

Food Eating Habits and Lifestyles 22

Tackling a Sugar Addiction 25

Conclusion 32

Author Bio 37

Publisher 48

Introduction

I was just browsing through one of the oh so clichéd books, which pass as escapist fiction today under the genre of chic-lit. And the female was suffering from He-Loves-Me-He-Loves-Me-Not blues, and that is why she went straight to the fridge, took out a large helping of ice cream, lots of chocolate, and had a really self pitying sob fest.

In the 21st-century, food is getting to be a psychological weapon, because psychologists are telling us that eating lots of it is going to give us a security blanket. This book is going to tell you all about how wrong they are, how unhealthy this addiction to food is, knowing more about a sugar addiction, and how you can wean yourself away from reaching for the nearest source of sugar and carbohydrates, whenever you feel like acting like a drama queen singing. *Nobody loves me. Everybody hates me I am going to the garden, to eat worms.*

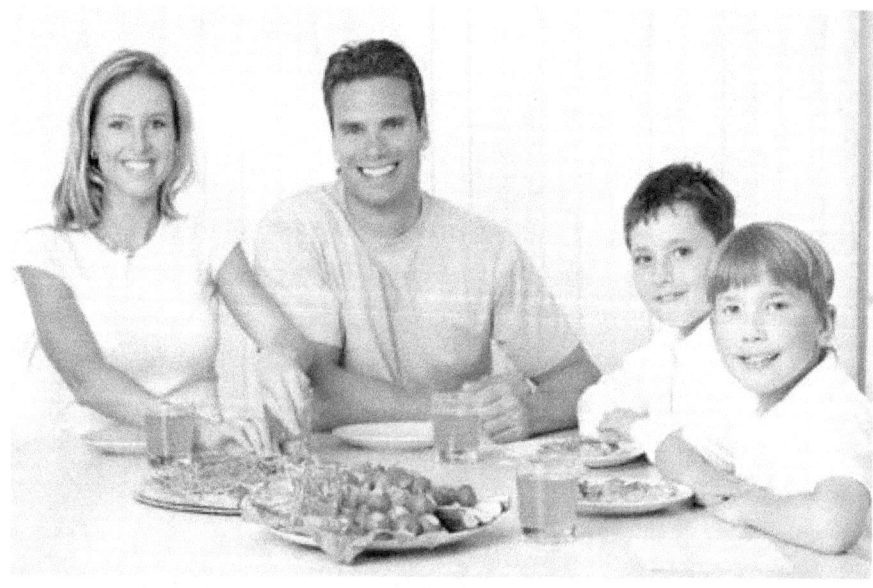

When youngsters start to appreciate healthy food, as children, they are going to remain healthy when they grow up to be adults.

This book is going to tell you all about how food can affect you psychologically, how it has been used as a comfort item, and how healthy eating can keep you spiritually, emotionally, physically, and mentally healthy.

Psychological Reasons for Unhealthy Eating Habits

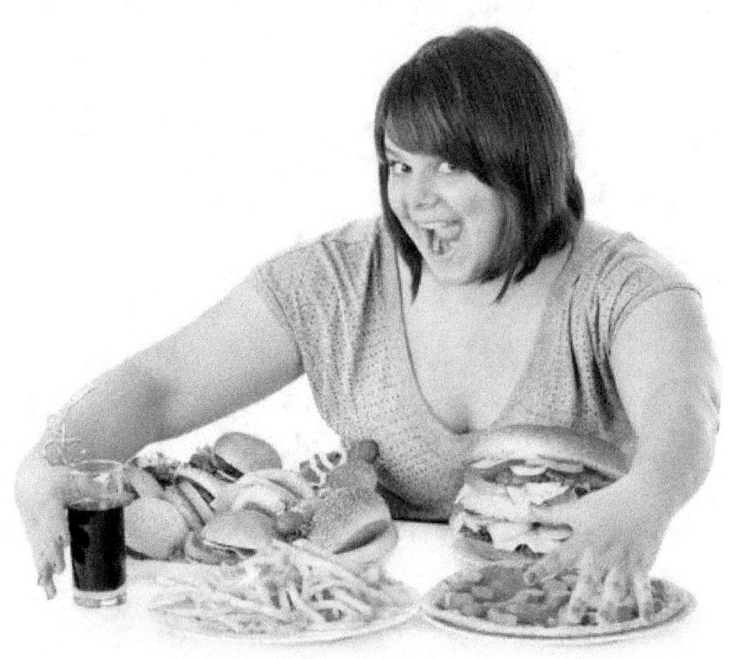

I went to a friend's house a couple of days ago and found her 25-year-old daughter, stuffing herself with lots of junk food. I took one look at that young girl, and not only did she look bloated, but she also looked pasty faced. Here was a young girl who had been once slim and slender, so this complete disregard towards a healthy diet made me wonder about the reason for this sudden craving for unhealthy and fat laden food.

When I laughingly asked her the reason for this extreme step, which made her eat and eat and eat, she told me soberly *that she did not have anything else to do.* In fact, she was so bored because she had had things too easily throughout her life. She was not allowed to do any job because her parents were so rich. She was sick and tired of doing the same things over and over again.

Apart from that, she had never been encouraged to cultivate any sort of constructive, positive strength. One could almost say that she had no spiritual resource or inner life to fall back upon.

When she was in her teens, she was very much in demand because she was an attractive young girl. But now that she had reached her 20s, she had nothing else to do except obsess about her weight and her looks. And she was so terribly fat, now that she was as one who was obsessed with fashion would say – frankly ugly. And no young man was going to look at her twice.

So what was she to do, the whole day long, but eat in order to pass her time.

Unfortunately, she has fallen prey to one of the 21st-century's most prevalent psychological problems – comfort foods.

Comfort Foods

This term was termed by a psychologist, somewhere in the 90s, who decided that there were a number of foods, which when eaten would give a mind, body, and spirit comfort, and this would include food items with lots of sugar content in it. Naturally, there was a scientific basis behind such a characteristic allocated to particular foods. All of them also had carbohydrates in them. And once you ate them, you just could not stop at one and continued eating them, on and on.

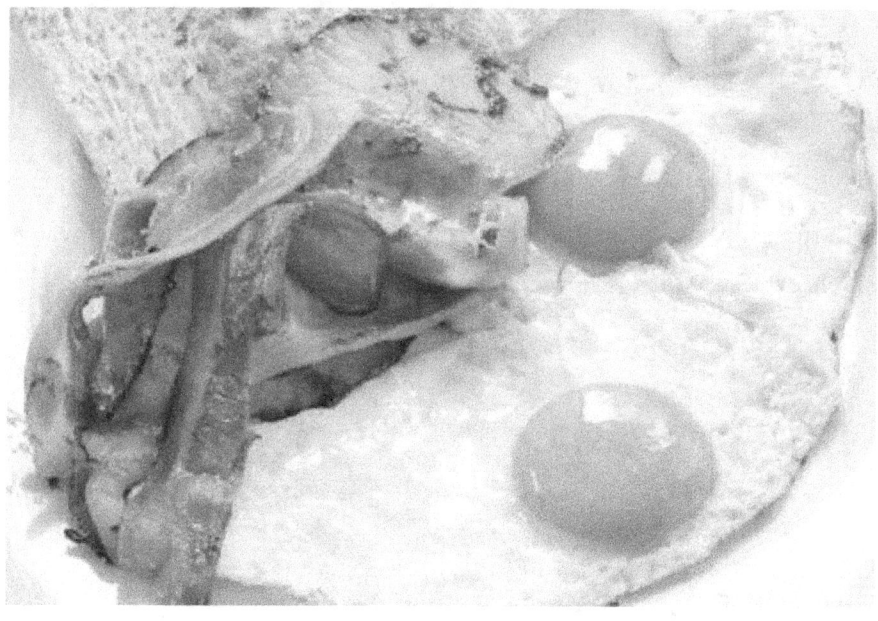

I do not know about you, but for me, a breakfast without bacon and eggs does not seem to be a fitting start to the day, also, hot buttered toast. For me, it is a comfort food, and once I have eaten this meal, I am ready to tackle anything, including hot weather and mosquitoes with equanimity.

Naturally, that was the first time when I heard this term so I went to one of psychologist friends and asked her to explain the psychology behind this eating, eating and eating.

Any sort of food which gives you psychological comfort is known as a comfort food. This is going to include chocolate, ice cream, and other calorie laden foods, which you do not eat normally in your daily diet. For a large number of people, this has become a sort of security blanket against any emotional hurt, any hiding away from reality or just because they are bored and they do not have anything constructive to do to while waiting for the time to pass.

So let us reach for something, right out of the fridge, to pass the time away.

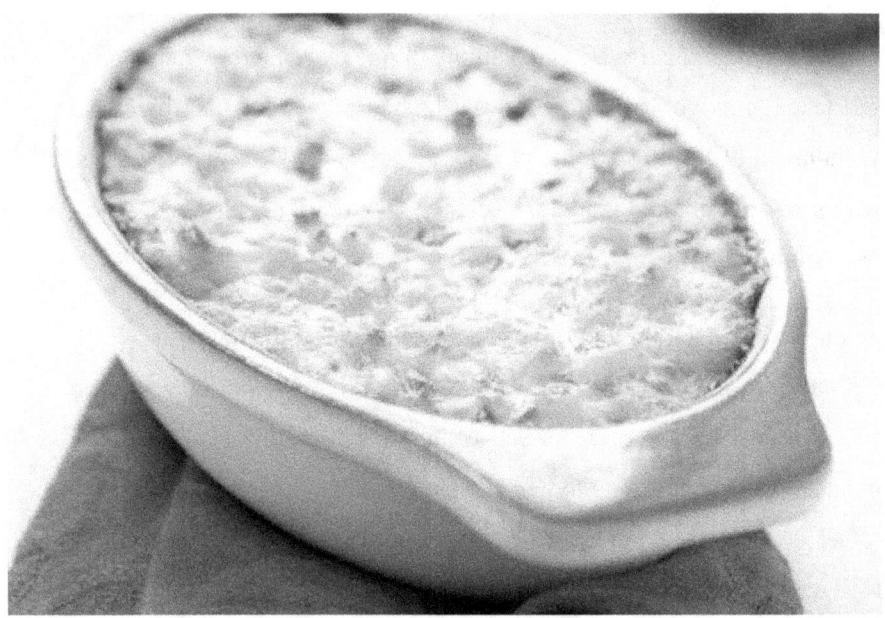

Comfort food is what people think we eat when we are sad or depressed. The deep-fried preparations, starches, and sugars satisfy this criteria, but the backlash takes the form of lethargy, melancholy, and of lots of weight gain. And so the downwards spiral gains momentum, with potentially unhealthy long-term effects.

Men associate hearty meals when they want comfort – thus, the terms – feed the brute and pacify him –, but women prefer snacks because there is also a feeling of guilt, associated with the knowledge that the foods which they are eating is not good for either their health or their figure. And naturally, they are right here.

Comfort food is actually sought out more when individuals are happy, jovial, and generally in celebratory times and as a reward for a job well done.

My friend's daughter was one example of one extreme to which a person can take the usage of comfort foods. She has this feeling that there was a withdrawal of affection of her parents towards her. This feeling can hit a person at any time in his life, especially when he is at a physical, spiritual, and emotional low.

Also, she had been brought up to do absolutely nothing constructive at all, with her life, except eat, drink, and be merry with no emotional support from parents, who were rather self-centered, selfish, and busy in their own personal lives. According to her, her parents could not care less about her future, even though they gave her plenty of money to compensate for the love and affection which she wanted.

So what else could she do, but spend the money on food, which supposedly gave her comfort throughout the day?

That reminded me of a friend of my mother's, about 60 years ago, who became a famous movie star of that time and married a director later on. However, at that time, being an actress was not considered to be a respectable profession, so her family kept ignoring the black sheep of the family, even though they did not mind all the expensive presents and gifts she sent her mother, father, and siblings in order to appease them and for forgiveness.

Her father was one of the richest men in the State. He had absolutely no time for his children, but every evening he used to come home, and throw bundles of notes on their beds, telling them that there was more coming, and they had to live life Emperor size. All they had to do was spend the money, and buy whatever they wished. This was 60 years ago! But apart from that, he could not care less about his family or their personal thoughts, or worries.

That girl decided that she had had enough of this sort of negligence, and she had better do something drastic in order to get some attention from her father. So she took the next train out to film land. Her father promptly disinherited her in typical melodramatic fashion and said that he had no daughter and she had lowered his name in the dust, and all that sort of clichéd jazz.

This young girl was talented, beautiful enough to get a job in films, as an extra, and then her director married her, because she had class, she had style, she belonged to a good family, and she definitely had self-respect and no way was she going to lower herself to be a part of the casting couch group.

And so she managed to gain some sort of respectability in the eyes of her father! Though of course he never supposedly forgave her for being such an undutiful daughter and not marrying the rich vice ridden alcoholic, he had chosen for her as a fitting groom.

Society has changed drastically, in the last 60 years, in the East, as well as in the West. Women have become more independent and have begun thinking for themselves. However, psychologically, they are still dependent on a large number of spiritual and emotional crutches and when they do not get them, they look for other options in order to get some sort of emotional satisfaction.

Collecting All Those Muffins

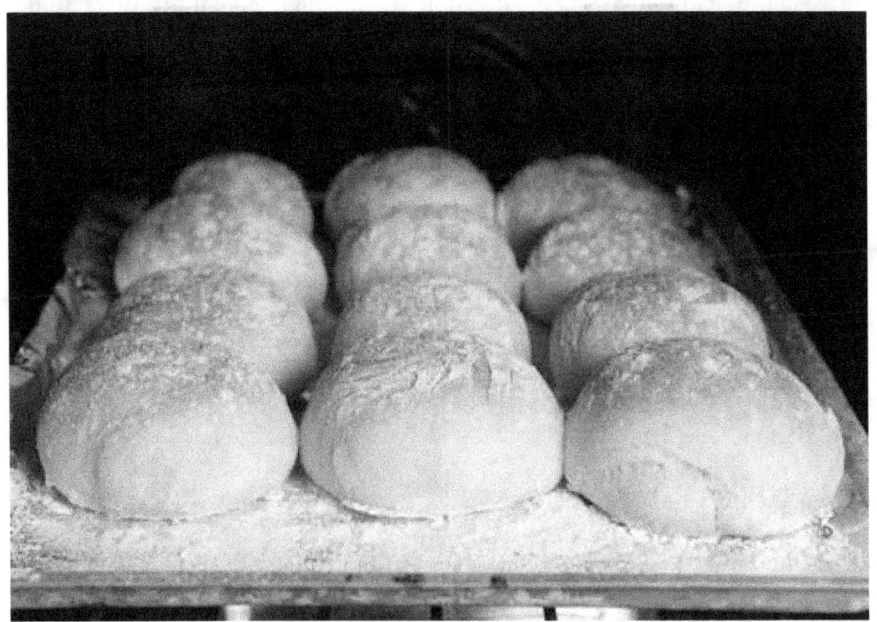

One day I overheard my father talking about a parable, which I think he had made up at the spur of the moment. I had a feeling that he was trying to get me to get rid of all the junk that I had accumulated in the house, during the past years, a side effect of raising a family and which I held dear, because of their emotional significance and memories.

There was a man who kept buying muffins every day. And he began to fill his house up with muffins. He never ate them, but his trunks were full up of muffins. So when he died, all one found were lots and lots of rooms, full of muffins, which he had never enjoyed during his lifetime, and saying that he would eat them one fine day. But that time never came, and he died without enjoying one single muffin.

And then he looked at me, as if asking me, if I understood anything about this illusion. And being a psychologist, I told him that it was clear that that man was trying to fill in some empty spaces within him, spiritual, emotional, or psychological with a physical, visible item, which gave him satisfaction and an emotional sort of comfort. And for him, muffins took that form. That man's psychological crutch was food, and the feeling that he could afford to buy enough muffins and would never go hungry again.

Father blinked, because this was too deep and involved a thought process for him, and possibly, he began to wonder what sort of spiritual, emotional, or psychological spaces, human beings had to fill in themselves, when they kept collecting lots and lots of things around them, even though they never used them at all? The metaphorical and symbolic muffins?

Not that I was spiritually, emotionally, or psychologically deprived or anything, I am too practical a person to be any of these things and would rather sit down and analyze the reason why I am feeling depressed, blue, or alternatively euphoric and content than go on a shopping or eating binge!

But, according to my father, my house was full of figurative muffins! As I grew older, I began throwing these "muffins" out, because I really did not want them and I really did not need them. This was the next stage of my spiritual and emotional growth, weaning myself away from childish things, I once held dear.

Now let us come to another aspect of food as a psychological weapon, especially in societies, where traditionally feeding the family was supposed to be the only way in which a mother could show how much she cared for her family.

Food As a Symbol of Love and Affection

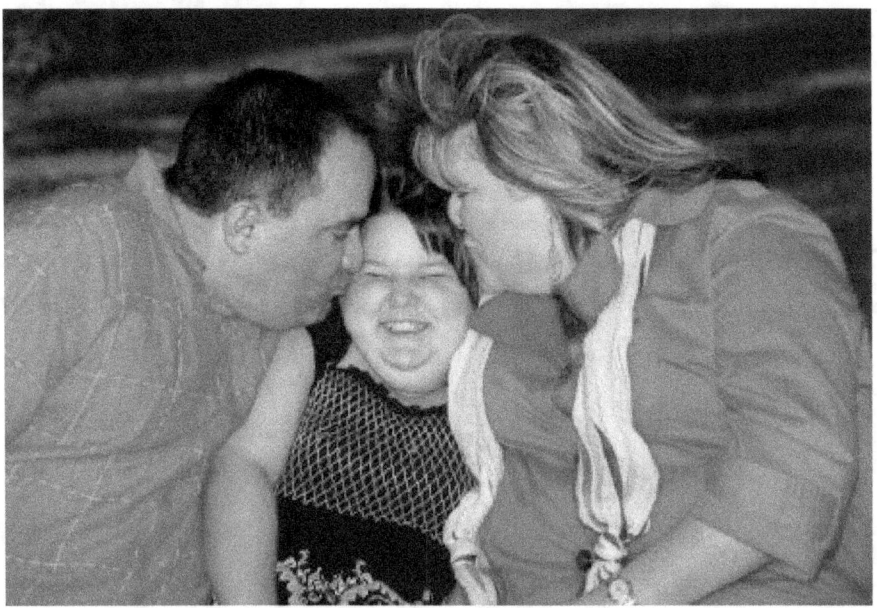

This is all very nice, but mom and dad have been feeding up their youngster a lot too!

How many times have you gone visiting friends, or acquaintances, and seeing them lovingly stuffing their children and family members with food? In many parts of the world, even today, feeding the family is directly associated with the amount of love and affection given by parents to their children. This comes down from prehistoric times, when only the rich and affluent could afford to have a regular three meals per day.

So the idea of having fat children or fat family members were directly related to the general prosperity of that particular family. Even today, in many parts of the East, a prosperous family is always described as a family which can eat and drink.

Well, let me give you my example. When we were kids, we were living in an area where all the children were brought up on a healthy, normal diet, then all of us were as healthy and thin as children could be and should be. This was in another part of the compass, which was culturally as different from my traditional cultural land and heritage as chalk from cheese.

So in summer, whenever we went to our native town to meet our relatives, the first thing they used to tell my father was – "look at the health of your children, could you not feed them up, they are as thin as bean poles. These children are starving" and other associated noises.

And then we used to be stuffed with all sorts of fattening and indigestible food, which had us suffering from indigestion and /or constipation within three days!

It was only later, when I grew up, and shifted back to my native town/land that I found out, that traditionally here, good eating and drinking was associated with a prosperous lifestyle. So, one had to be fat in order to be considered attractive, of a good family, and prosperous enough to eat whatever one wanted, whenever one wanted, and as often as one could!

Naturally, that is how, traditionally, great-grandmothers, grandmothers and mothers had imbibed the notion that the best way to show a caring attitude towards family members was to feed them, feed them often, and feed them well!

This attitude is not just restricted to the East. I have seen it in Italy and Spain, where mamas love feeding their daughters and sons, and even guests with really delicious and tasty home-cooked meals. They get really offended if you say no to second and third helpings! Here, they are being a universal mother again, and are doing exactly what the sisterhood of mothers have been doing for millenniums all over the world, be it Italy, Spain, Egypt, America, Japan, China, or any other country of which you could think, where good meals are appreciated!

No wonder anybody going to Italy or Spain should forget about a diet, because of the good and delicious food available there in large quantities which cannot be resisted, especially when there is somebody to cajole you into taking another helping, while saying you need some fat on your bones!

So now, this is not a matter of comfort food being fed to you, but more of an extension of a feminine and motherly version of maternal love. In some way, you can say that she is comforting herself knowing that her family has been well fed!

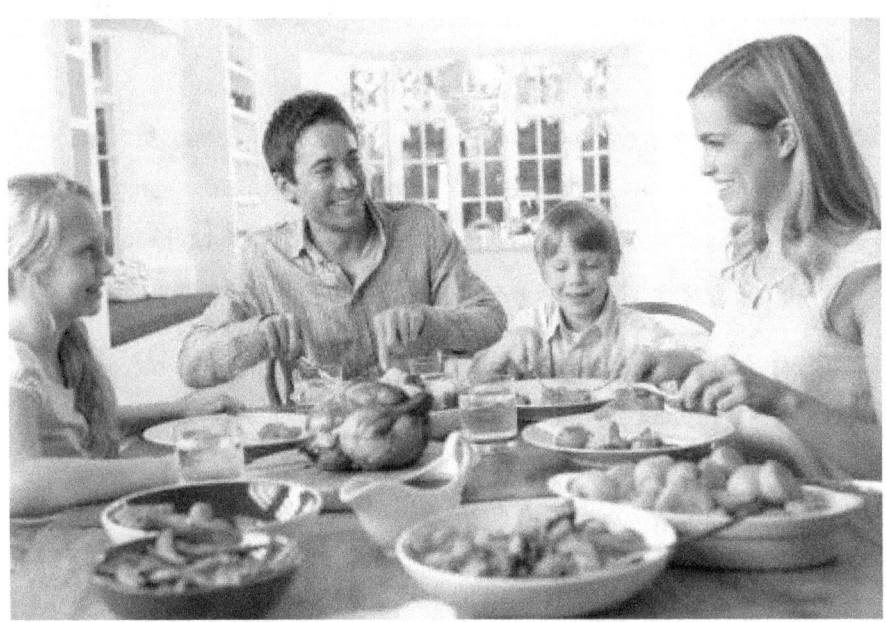

A well fed family is a happy family. It is also going to be an obese one. Especially when children are given full leeway to eat what they want, and whenever they want.

Using food as a substitute to show love, or using it as a comfort food item for the deprivation of love – both of these are activities which are deeply rooted and psychological traits. And that is why down the ages food has always been associated with being the best way to someone's heart. And now it is being used to comfort someone who feels that the people around him do not have any heart!

So what are the positive points of indulging in comfort foods? Well, they make you feel good because you have got a little more glucose in your system.

On the other hand, psychological eating disorders like anorexia, bulimia, and overeating take place when a person thinks he can only keep someone's love, respect, and affection by being extremely slim or gaining attention by getting fat and bloated.

Remember that the psychological tricks do not work. A person I know decided to get back at the parents, she loved, but who she thought were not paying her enough attention, but all their time, money, energy, and everything else was being spent, according to her on her siblings.

Now this girl can be considered to be plenty selfish and self-centered, depending on which psychologist has her under his care, but on the other hand, parental pressure can also have a lot of negative subconscious psychological effect on your psyche.

The parents liked her and their children well groomed, exquisitely turned out every moment of the day so that they could be a credit to them in society! That particular friend of mine reached the stage when she found herself to be a puppet performing on a stage with everybody applauding her general appearance from Cinderella to Princess with the parents taking all the credit and the totally narcissistic mother telling everybody that yes, she knew that she looked young enough to be the sister of her kids!

When a person reaches this stage when she feels that she is not love for herself alone, but because she is the extension of someone else, she is usually going to turn to comfort food for emotional and spiritual support.

Now remember, this complete revulsion of feeling is what parents have to guard against. On the other hand do not overburden your child with love, which is harmful for him and that also includes showing your love by feeding him or her continuously.

Believe it or not, this is a part and parcel of the human existence, all over the world, and has been so for millenniums. Even today, my mother wants me to be the perfect daughter, and sometimes, it is very painful, visiting her at her house, because one knows that one will have to bear the brunt of eagle eyed parental scrutiny, and adverse criticism of – good Lord, what are you wearing, look at your hair, look at your skin, what have you been doing to yourself, why don't you lose some weight, you used to be so smart and well turned out – 25/30 years ago, when I was 25/30 years younger and needed to be well groomed due to the demands of my job/profession – and blah blah blah.

No wonder, whenever I go visit her, I want to cut my journey short and get back home, as fast as possible. I never stay with her for more than one night and that is much more than enough for about a year or so!

And while I am there, I raid the fridge for ice cream and something fattening, just because! If a responsible, professionally and personally successful, self-confident person like I can be turned into this state of quivering inferiority, and depression, I wonder about the state of children not tough enough to bear the arrows and slings of continuous parental disapproval and criticism, 24/7!

On the other hand do not have such a disinterested and unattached attitude towards your child by thinking that material riches that you gave him are more than enough and can take the place of an emotional and spiritual bond between parent and child.

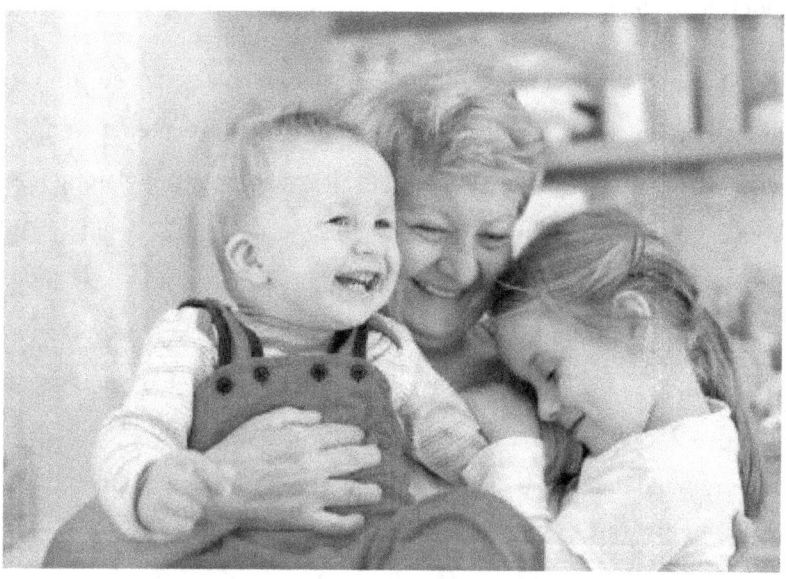

Grandmas are for spoiling! Just the feeling that there is grandma there to hug and hold you and laugh with you, and give you undemanding love is quite enough to make a child feel happy, content, and secure. Best of all, grandma knows what you like to eat, and she makes it for you! With all natural and healthy ingredients!

Remember as parents, you have to be very careful about the thin red line between overindulgence and apathy. A once healthy and happy child can suddenly feel that his parents really would not care less about him and so he is going to start snacking on comfort foods. This is one easy item, which can be bought with all that pocket money you have been showering upon him.

Food Eating Habits and Lifestyles

Remember, that the 21st-century concept of healthy eating is – if you really care about the health of your family, remember that the idea of an excellent housewife, or mother is one who feeds her family well, but in a healthy manner.

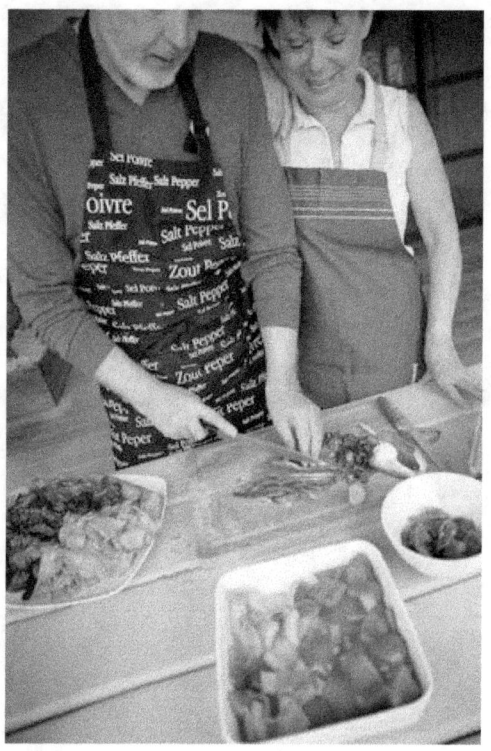

The day of showing how loving and caring you are by feeding them well and feeding them often is a bit outdated now. The welfare family idea was acceptable in the times – ancient and medieval, when only prosperous people could afford three solid meals a day, as I said before.

The poor women who could afford only one meal a day for their families tried their best to make it so nourishing and tasty because it had to last out until the next meal, which would either be easily available or perhaps there would be an interim of starvation until this food or materials could be obtained for another nourishing meal.

That is why they used totally natural products like herbs, vegetables, fruit, nuts, and other bounties of nature in order to make up a good meal. I remember my grandmother telling me a story which her grandmother had told her. They came from a village area, where life was hard, and times were hard. However, keeping up with Eastern tradition, the idea of hospitality to family members and guests was a sacred concept, and had to be followed.

So my grandmother's grandmother as a new bride asked her mother in law, how she should cope when unexpected guests in the shape of relatives turned up, one fine evening, as hungry as bears, and expected food.

Taking the timescale, this must have been about 150 – 200 years ago and that lady had got this knowledge from her ancestors!

So here it goes – if you belong to a good family and you can give them meat, put water in the meat, and give them bread and gravy. Fill up the empty spaces with buttermilk. If you can afford only pulses and lentils, put potatoes in the pulses, and make gravy of onions, tomatoes, and spices and herbs. And then add enough water not to make a watery gravy, but a delicious potato lentil soup with lots of bread and buttermilk.

Naturally, these were the shifts to which, these ladies were used to feed their family members every day, day in, day out on limited budgets and supplies.

In fact, my grandmother never left the cooking of the bread to the cook. That was the woman of the house's prerogative so that she could regulate the intake of the food being eaten by each and every family member depending on how long the supplies lasted and how much she wanted to feed them!

And after the meal was done, she always put one piece of bread in the bread box, wrapped up in a piece of cloth. When I asked her that we had already finished our meal, and what was that bread for, she said that this was traditional. Because the breadbox would never be empty if it had something in it, and sometimes that piece of bread would come in useful to feed anybody who felt hungry at any time! And also, when a guest came, and came into the kitchen, looking for something to eat, the first thing he would do was open the breadbox.

If there was something there, he would psychologically be reassured that there was enough food, because one piece of bread was going waste, according to him, because you could see it in the breadbox.

Grandmother used to crumble that piece of bread, the next morning and feed them to the birds and squirrels, crows, sparrows, and pigeons in the garden. They loved her very much and she only had to open the door and say *come come come*, for them to come flying for their breakfast.

Well, these are glimpses into times and ages gone past, but they are psychologically indications of how people lived all those years ago.

And now I come to another major important part of our eating habits in the 21st century – the craving for sugar.

Tackling a Sugar Addiction

It is true, men and women both suffer from a sweet tooth. That is because any healthy human brain, regardless of it belonging to a man or a woman has to produce a hormone named dopamine to keep functioning naturally.

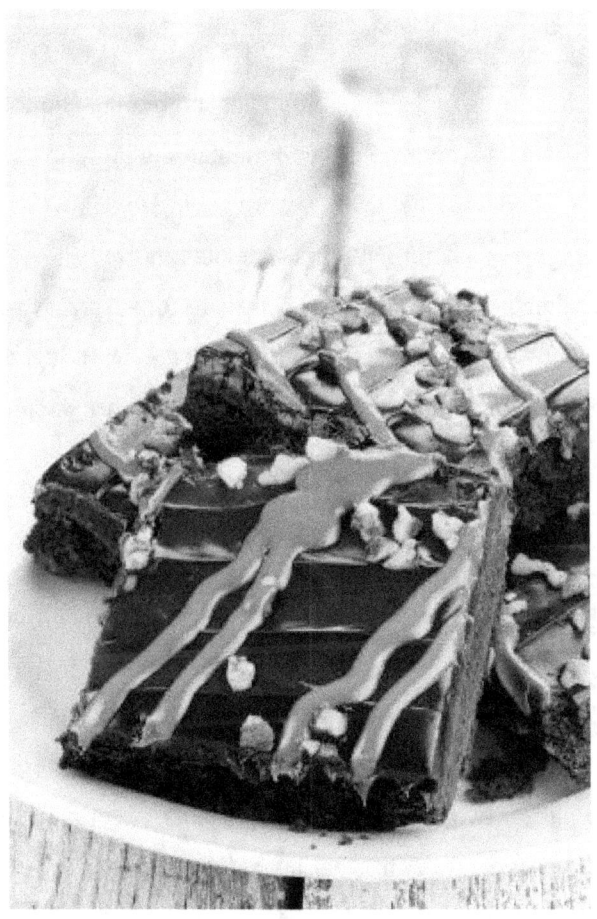

Did you know that 62% of the people all around the world are suffering from a sugar addiction? You do not believe it. This trend has escalated in the

21st-century, especially when in ancient times, people did not have access to enough of sugar in large enough quantities to make them addicted to it.

But with the coming of modern technology, and refining processes giving you plenty of access to plenty of sugary products, is it a surprise that you are suffering from a sweet tooth?

You just cannot resist eating anything sugary. In fact, you have this craving for something sugary and sweet, especially after your meals.

I remember when I was undergoing my teachers training about 12 years ago in a school, in an area where we did communicating more in the vernacular than in English. And one fine day, we were having lunch, when one of fellow teachers just came out with this statement in English – "every evening, after dinner, my husband has a craving for sugar." Now this word craving was something very unexpected from her, even though she pronounced it "crabing," but everybody understood what she meant! And then she added, "He has a sweet tooth. And so I have it, too."

So after dinner, each night, they walked one and a half miles to one of the city's well-known traditional sweetshop to have just *one piece of traditionally made coconut sweet – meat* each, and then walked back again, the hunger for something sweet appeased for the day.

I found that very interesting psychologically speaking. Why not half? Why not one and a half or two? Why just that particular sweet meat? And when I asked her the reason why she had not taken her choice of any other sweet meats, she just shrugged her shoulders and said that particular quantity suited her and her husband just fine!

Well, she had her craving for sugar well under control. And a 3 mile walk after dinner kept them both fit and fine.

But how many of us have the time and energy and inclination to go walking after dinner, especially after we have gotten rid of that sugar – craving with delicious puddings, pies, and custards?

Believe it or not, according to the Worldwide Health Organization (WHO), 1.9 billion people worldwide are overweight, with 600 million of them considered seriously obese and that is because of excess sugar consumption. This has contributed directly to that gain in weight.

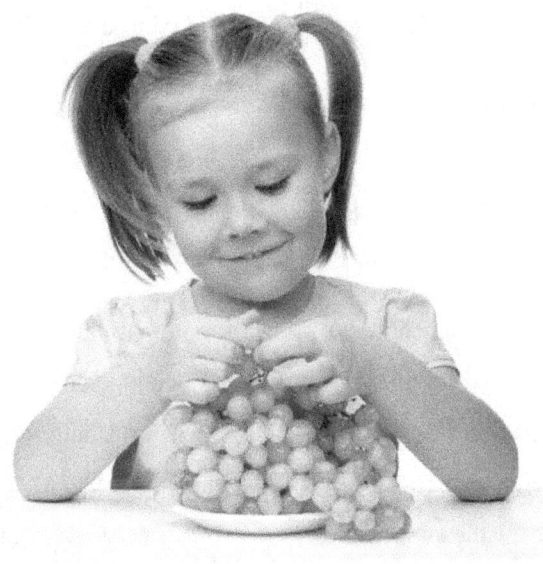

Every living thing needs a bit of sugar to keep working in a healthy fashion. So get your sugar high from natural fruit.

Apart from this, scientists have proven that some particular areas of the brain are controlled by dopamine. This gives you a feeling of euphoria. High consumption of sugar is going to elevate the levels of dopamine and that means the portions of the brain, which make you feel emotions like happiness, pleasure and so on are affected.

Incidentally, this stimulation is equal to the stimulation given to you by a number of drugs, especially recreational drugs like tobacco, morphine, and cocaine!

Surprising isn't it, that the idea of being addicted to cocaine and morphine makes us shudder, but the idea of an addiction to sugar leaves us supremely unmoved! That is how selective brainwashing has been done to us by companies who do not want to tell us that eating their excessive sugary products are quite capable of getting us addicted to that stuff.

Incidentally, this reminds me of my childhood, when a sugar cotton candy man posted himself just outside our school premises, and at lunchtime, all of us made a beeline for him to get our fix of sugar candy, incidentally, spending all our pocket money on that pink candy fluff.

Those who did not have enough of pocket money to buy the fluff kept asking their friends for a bite of that sticky delectable gooey material! Luckily, our teachers were sensible enough to know that there was something drastically wrong happening somewhere, when all the children made a beeline for the sugar candy man and our principal told him to take himself off.

Believe it or not, all of us 126 schoolchildren began suffering from sugar candy withdrawal, and I still remember our feeling of discomfort, bad temper, bad mood, lethargy, and other physical reactions which of course we were too young to understand and accept.

Incidentally, that had such an effect on me, that I stopped eating sugary stuff altogether, and even today, I eat any sweet item very rarely. And that is why

I can say I do not suffer from a weight problem or a bad temper dopamine levels drop off problem.

Because, when you are getting addicted to sugar, you are going to feel euphoric in the initial stages. But continuous and long-term consumption of sugar is going to lead to the reduction of the levels of dopamine being produced in your brain.

This means that you are going to eat more sugar to get the same level of pleasurable, euphoria, and good cheer.

Also, it is a well-known fact that if you get addicted to sugar in your childhood, and eat lots of it, and as often as possible, you are going to follow a pattern of binge eating when you grow up. You are going to suffer from psychiatric and neurological problems and consequences which are going to affect your emotional moods and physical well-being.

Scientists say that, today. I am not a degree waving scientist, but I said it before.

Believe it or not, in the USA, drugs, which have been approved by the FDA, which have been used to treat nicotine addiction – Champix – is being used to treat sugar addictions. That is because the symptoms produced by both these addictions have the same bio physiological effect on your mind.

So the next time you begin to think that you want something sweet to eat, sit back, and wonder why you have this sudden craving for sugar. Did somebody tell you that it was necessary and nodded to keep your glucose levels high? Are you so exhausted/tired and lethargic that you need an artificial boost of energy and want to dope up on Dopamine?

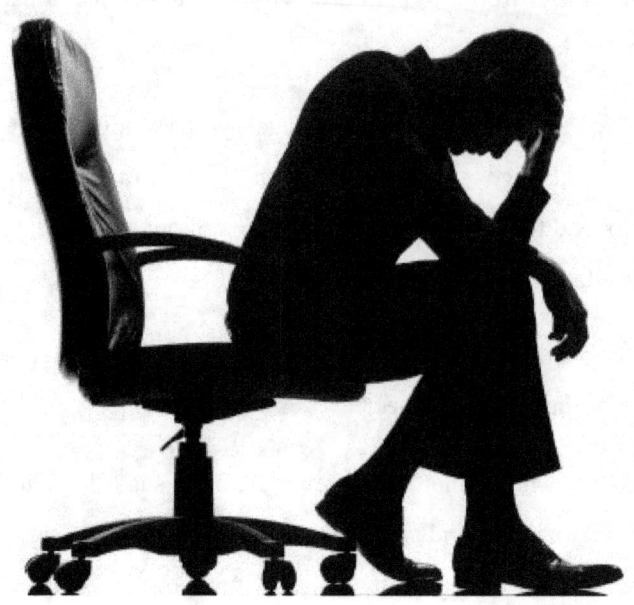

Why can't I seem to concentrate and think properly? I need something.

Consider, think, and slowly begin weaning yourself away from sugar. Naturally, you are going to suffer from withdrawal symptoms, because you are not getting your high of good cheer without that lump of sugar. But think of its benefits. No weight problems, no possible chances of diabetes, and best of all, no long-term after effects of going into depression because that sudden craving for sugar could not be fixed.

In ancient times, the sugar content needed by a body was supplied through fruit, honey, beetroot sugar, maple, and sugarcane sugar. All of these were natural products and were eaten in just small quantities.

Nowadays, we have so many types of sugars available to us, including that terrible unhealthy corn syrup, and refined sugar granules. And so many tempting items all around us, which have sugars as preservatives like jams, jellies, and marmalades. No wonder most of us are suffering from sugar addiction.

So incidentally, if the next time you feel lethargic and not so energetic and somebody just hands you a piece of chocolate, try this alternative instead – just take a glass of fresh fruit juice. It is going to prevent dehydration, it is going to give you enough sugar and in a natural form to prevent you from feeling mentally low and depressed and best of all, your dopamine levels are not going to be fussed around with, manipulated, or influenced artificially.

Conclusion

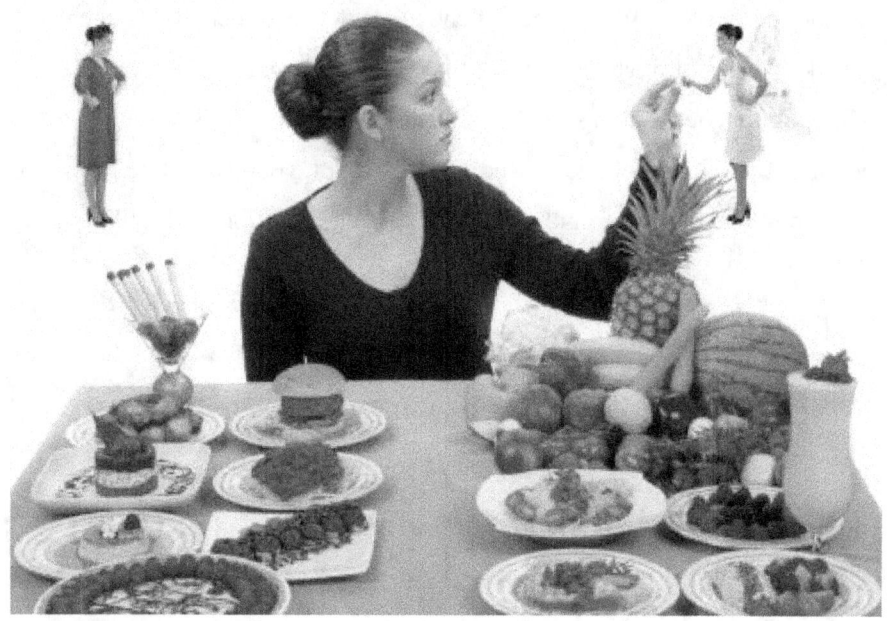

This book has given you plenty of information about food as a psychological weapon, and the historical, physiological, spiritual, and emotional significance behind using food as a psychological weapon, especially as a comfort food.

But remember, food has been an integral part of our lives, for millenniums, especially good food and drink, and one of mankind's main reasons for leaving was the pursuit of good food and drink to enjoy.

Nevertheless, there were times when mankind did not have food in large quantities, ready at hand. We in the 21st-century are luckier in this respect that we have plenty of choices of food, right at hand, but unfortunately we have forgotten the premier rule of existence – an excess of everything is going to give you access of trouble later on in life!

As that is why most of us with our changed lifestyles find ourselves obsessing about our weight, our terrible looking skin, our unhealthy physiques, our state of general bad health and blame everybody and everything around us, except the main culprit – our hunger for lots and lots of food, even when we do not need to eat it.

But then, man has forgotten another important rule – A Sensible Man Eats to Live and Does Not Live to Eat. But as time went by, every civilization evolved its own particular cuisine, depending on the availability of the foods available to the people at that time, and how it could be made appetizing, good to look at, and nourishing as well as delicious and filling.

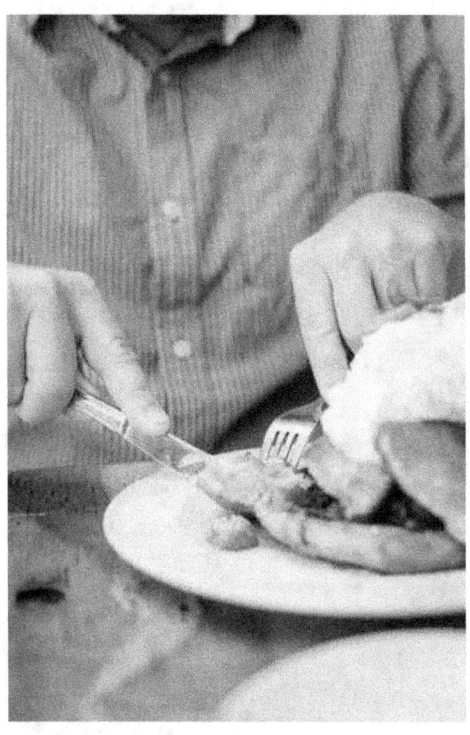

In ancient times, let us say ancient Rome, the priests used to get the first choice of food items sacrifice to the Gods in the temples. After that came the rich people and after that came the poor, to which the priests sold the hooves, offal, and other supposedly worth – discarding parts to the common people, and that is why the mothers of Rome had to look for the best ways in which this unappetizing fare could be turned into something nourishing and delicious for their brood.

That is why their cuisine evolved in something so unique, with the judicial use of herbs – they could not afford spices – along with vegetables and seasonings, like dried fish, onions, garlic, and other herbs.

And Rome survived for three millenniums on onions, garlic, bread, salt, and garum, which was an anchovy sauce. And the Romans did not starve. Even at that time, the concept of feeding a family well, and in just enough of portions, which would keep the family healthy and going strong, was well known to the family cook.

Naturally, this was also known to other peoples of other lands, who had to make do with items they had at hand. And that is why the idea of indulging in lots of food was restricted only to those self-indulgent hedonistic types who really did not have anything constructive to do with their time and spent it in the art of gastronomy and fine eating and drinking.

So remember the whole concept about feeding a family well and keeping it happy can now be seen by aviation mothers and housewives as following the same principle, but the food is going to be in smaller portions and helpings!

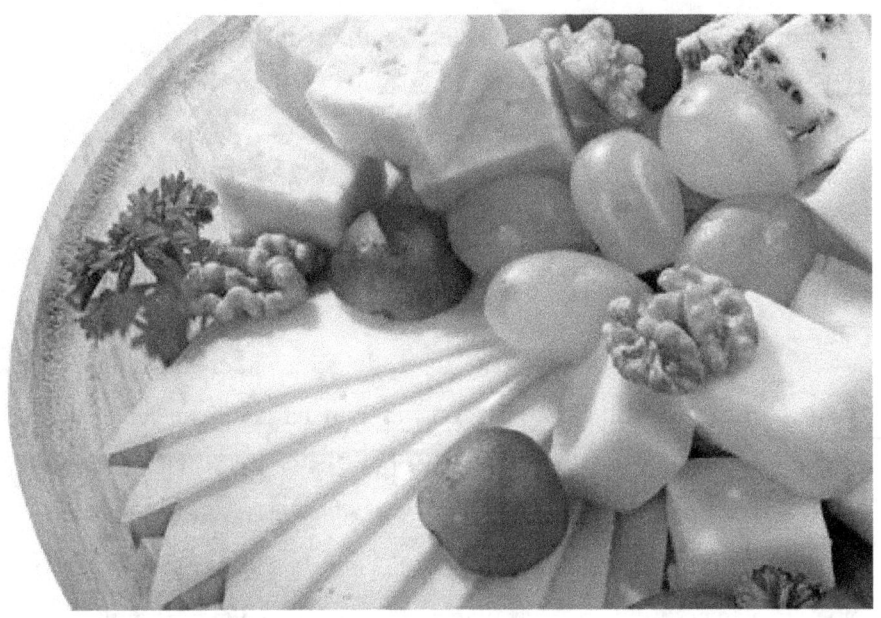

Natural, healthy food in small portions is a much better choice than lots and lots of food on an overstocked plate.

So if you are following the ingrained habit of breakfast, brunch, lunch, snacks, high tea, dinner, and then afterwards something else, and stuff your family as much as you can, after all you love them so much do not you and you are a good, caring, loving mother, are not you, take a breather and step back!

Please do not make the mistake of imagining that it can ever compensate for any emotional ties, whether they are of love or just plain disinterest. And remember the next time that you are extremely gloomy and sad and reach for the nearest sweet food or salty food for comfort, stop, look, and remember. Food can never be a security blanket, though it is something to chew on, and keep you busy for a little while.

If you are using food as a shelter against pain, trouble, and the burden of life which you are undergoing, just like intoxicants, comfort food can also be addictive. And soon you are going to reach this stage when you don't care less about your surroundings, your reality, your future, your present but more about your fix which makes you feel better and that is food. Incidentally, it is adding all those extra inches to your hips.

Instead, you may try listening to music, reading a book, or watching a funny movie. If you really want to nibble something, reach for some bean sprouts, fruit, or raw vegetables. If you want something salty on them, just cut them up, sprinkle a little bit of salt and pepper on them – some seasoned salt, which is a healthy option like garlic and celery salt, rock salt, black salt, and some dried spices mixture, seasoning and enjoy. No feelings of guilt, you have found something to chew upon while listening to music or reading a book. Isn't that comforting enough?

So take comfort from your food, but only if it is nourishing you and not being a substitute for something else! Live Long and Prosper!

Author Bio

Dueep Jyot Singh is a Management and IT Professional who managed to gather Postgraduate qualifications in Management and English and Degrees in Science, French and Education while pursuing different enjoyable career options like being an hospital administrator, IT,SEO and HRD Database Manager/ trainer, movie , radio and TV scriptwriter, theatre artiste and public speaker, lecturer in French, Marketing and Advertising, ex-Editor of Hearts On Fire (now known as Solstice) Books Missouri USA, advice columnist and cartoonist, publisher and Aviation School trainer, ex-moderator on Medico.in, banker, student councilor ,travelogue writer … among other things!

One fine morning, she decided that she had enough of killing herself by Degrees and went back to her first love -- writing. It's more enjoyable! She already has 48 published academic and 14 fiction- in- different- genre books under her belt.

When she is not designing websites or making Graphic design illustrations for clients , she is browsing through old bookshops hunting for treasures, of which she has an enviable collection – including R.L. Stevenson, O.Henry, Dornford Yates, Maurice Walsh, De Maupassant, Victor Hugo, Sapper, C.N. Williamson, "Bartimeus" and the crown of her collection- Dickens "The Old Curiosity Shop," and "Martin Chuzzlewit" and so on… Just call her "Renaissance Woman" - collecting herbal remedies, acting like Universal Helping Hand/Agony Aunt, or escaping to her dear mountains for a bit of exploring, collecting herbs and plants, and trekking.

Check out some of the other JD-Biz Publishing books

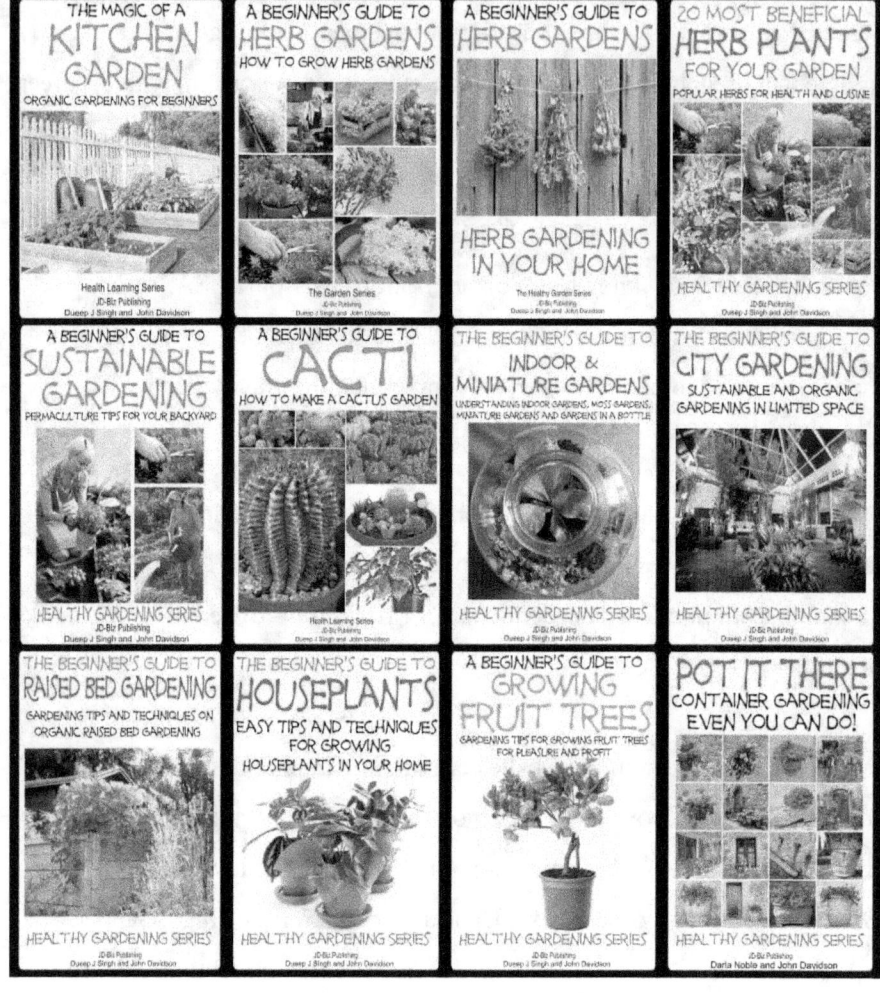

Health Learning Series

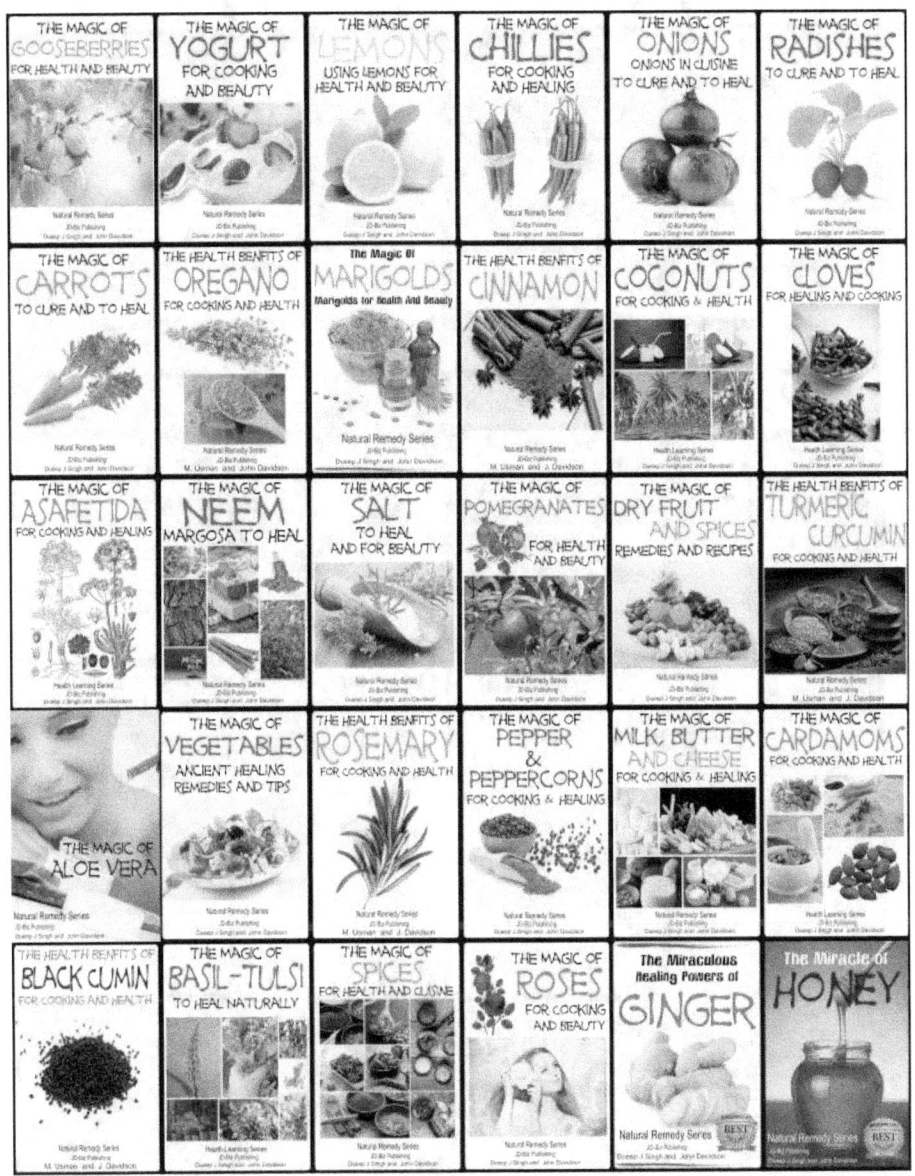

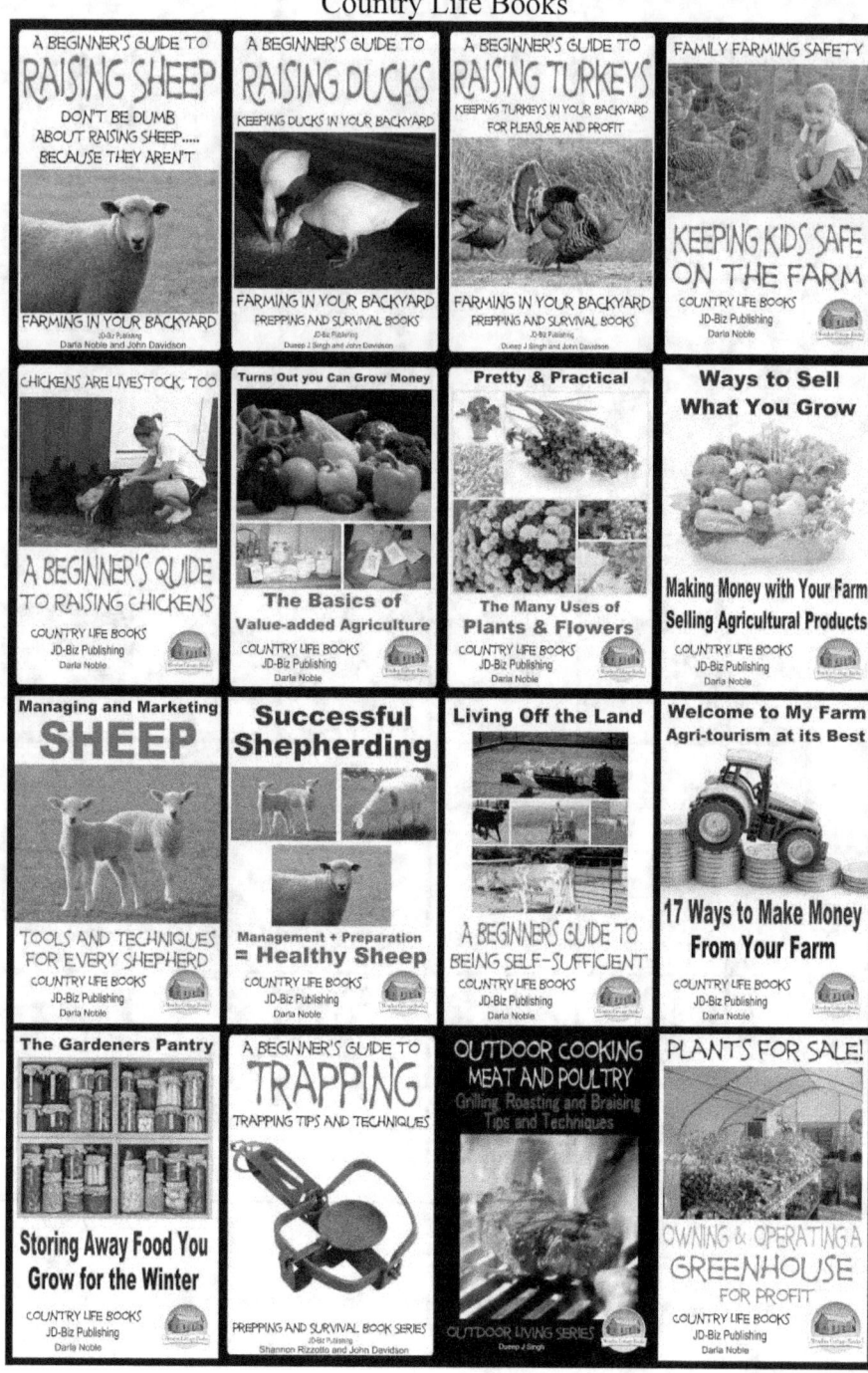

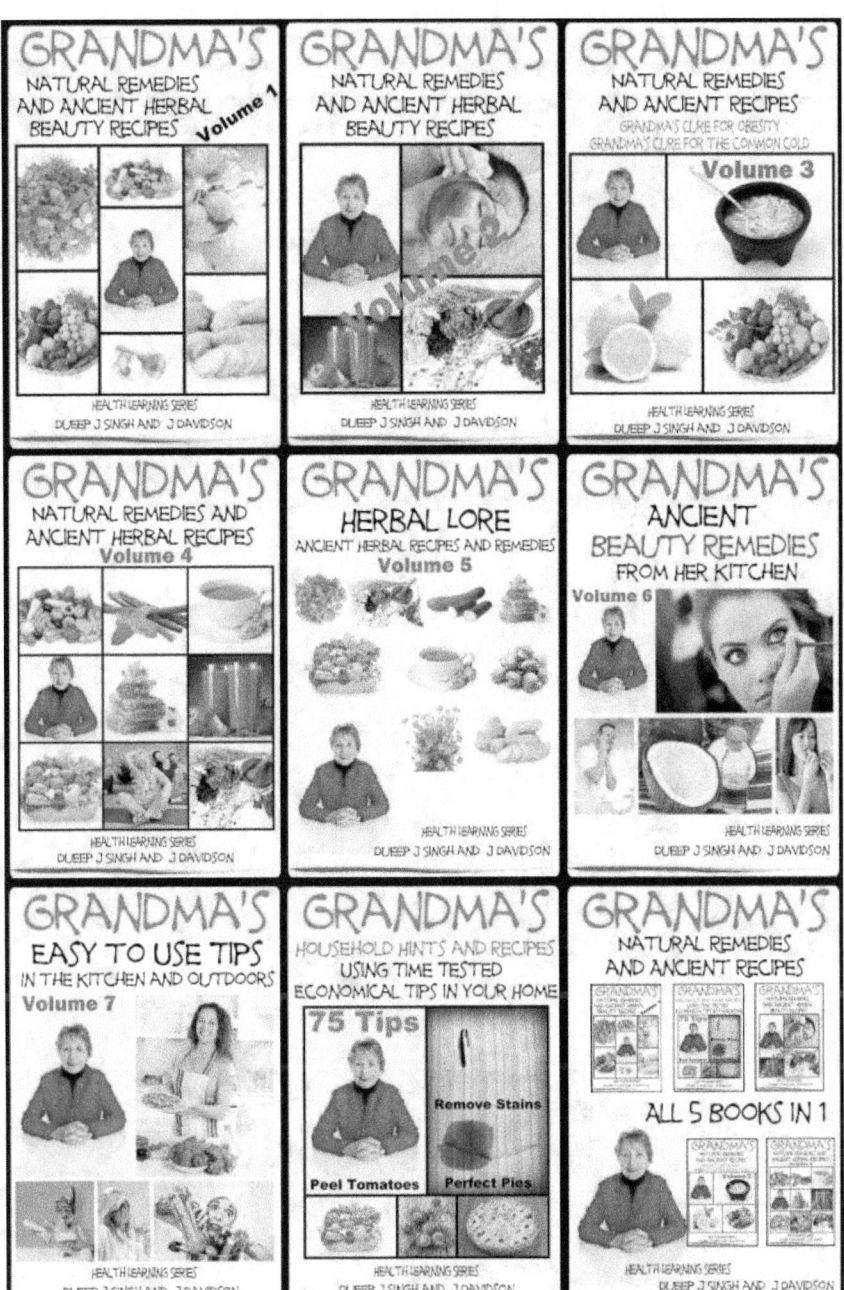

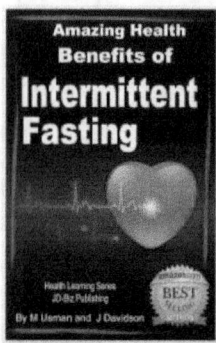
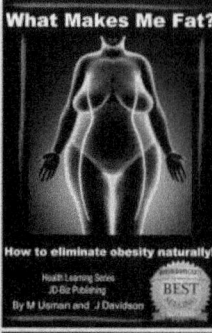
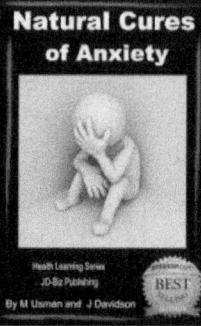
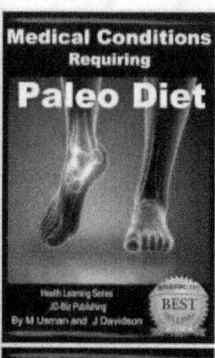
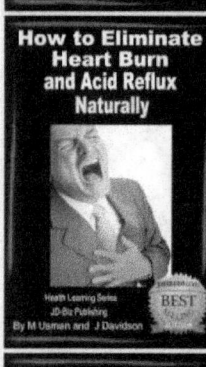
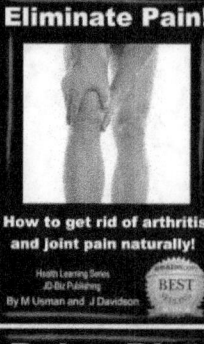
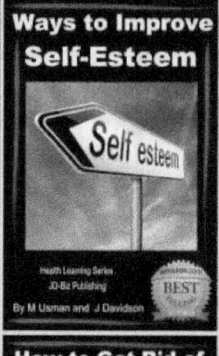
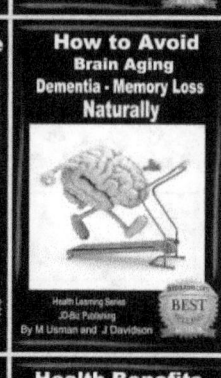
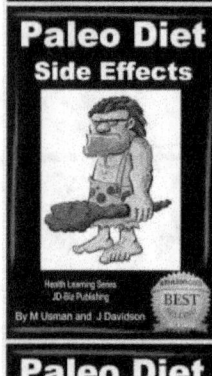
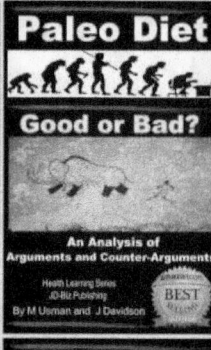
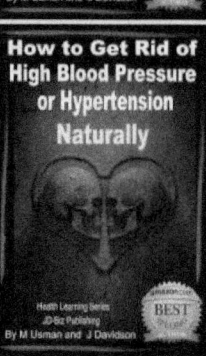
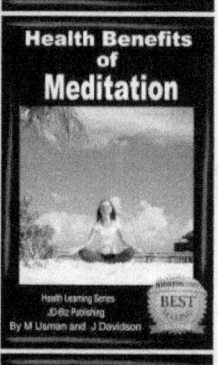
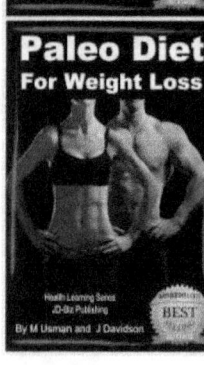
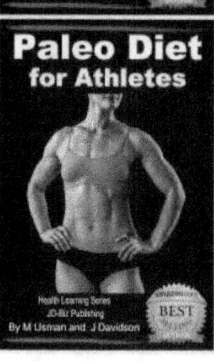
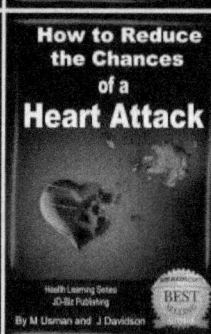
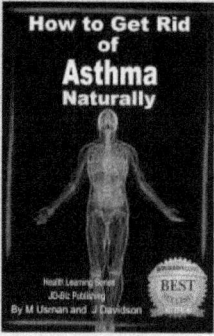

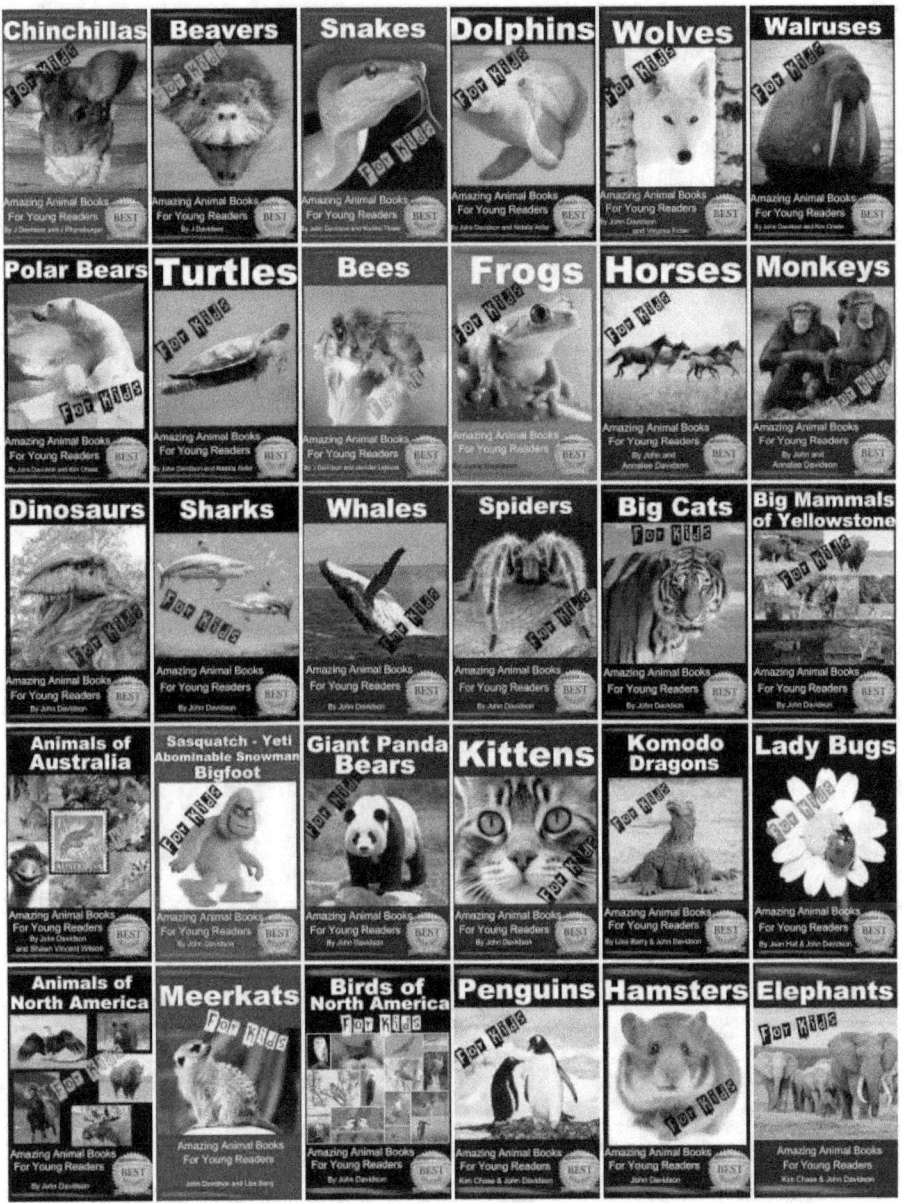

Learn To Draw Series

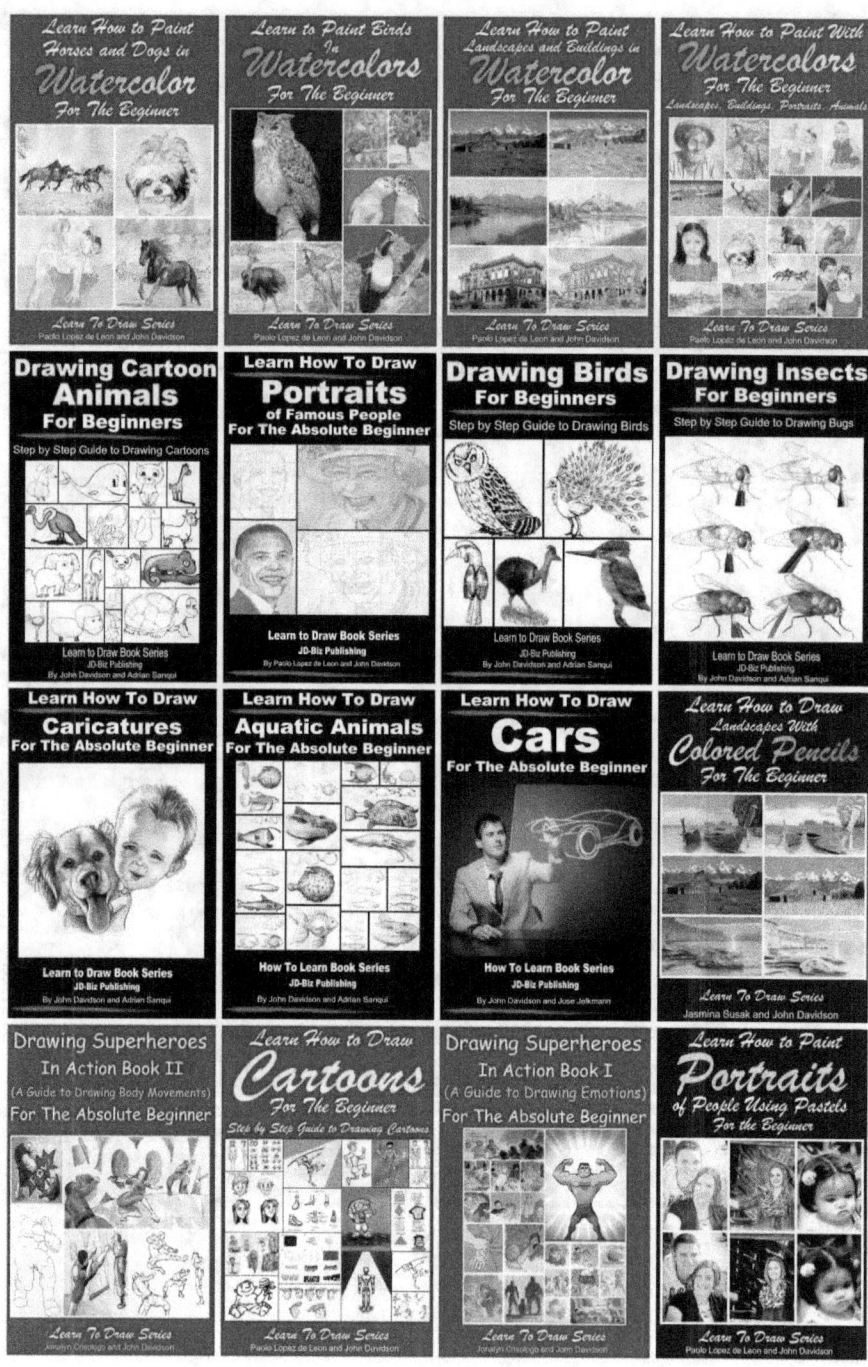

How to Build and Plan Books

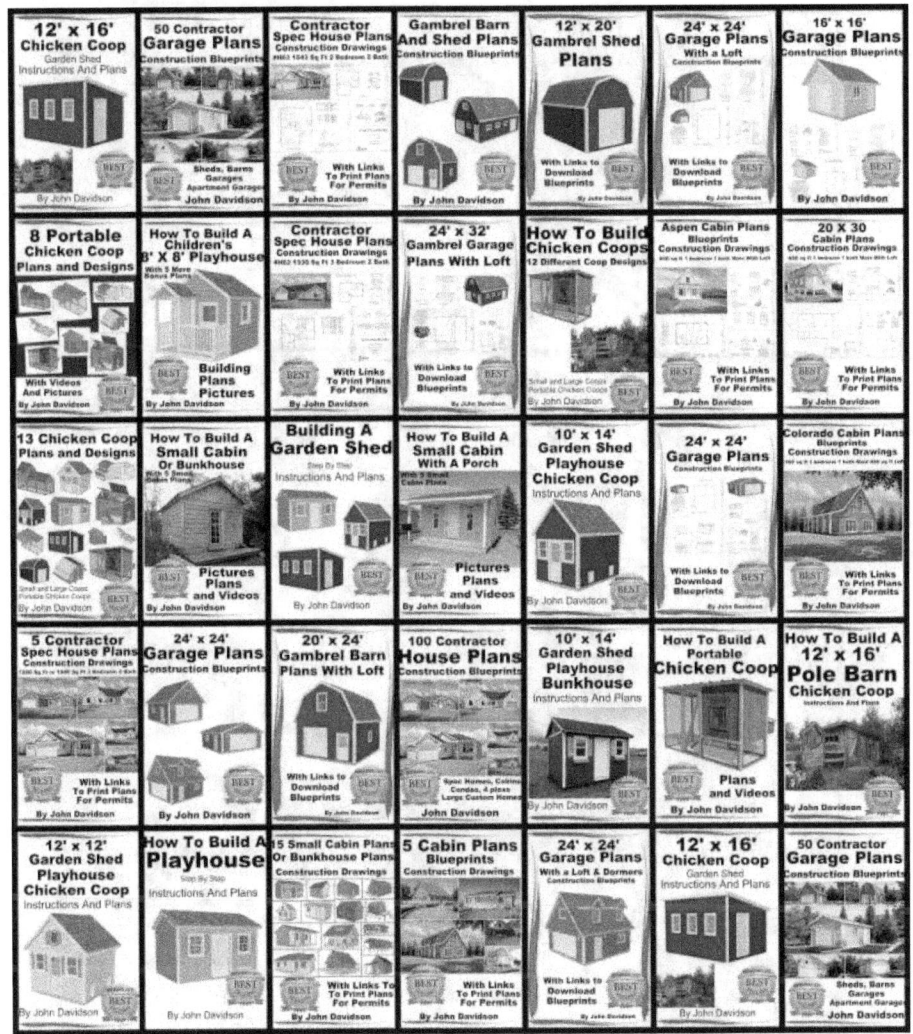

Entrepreneur Book Series

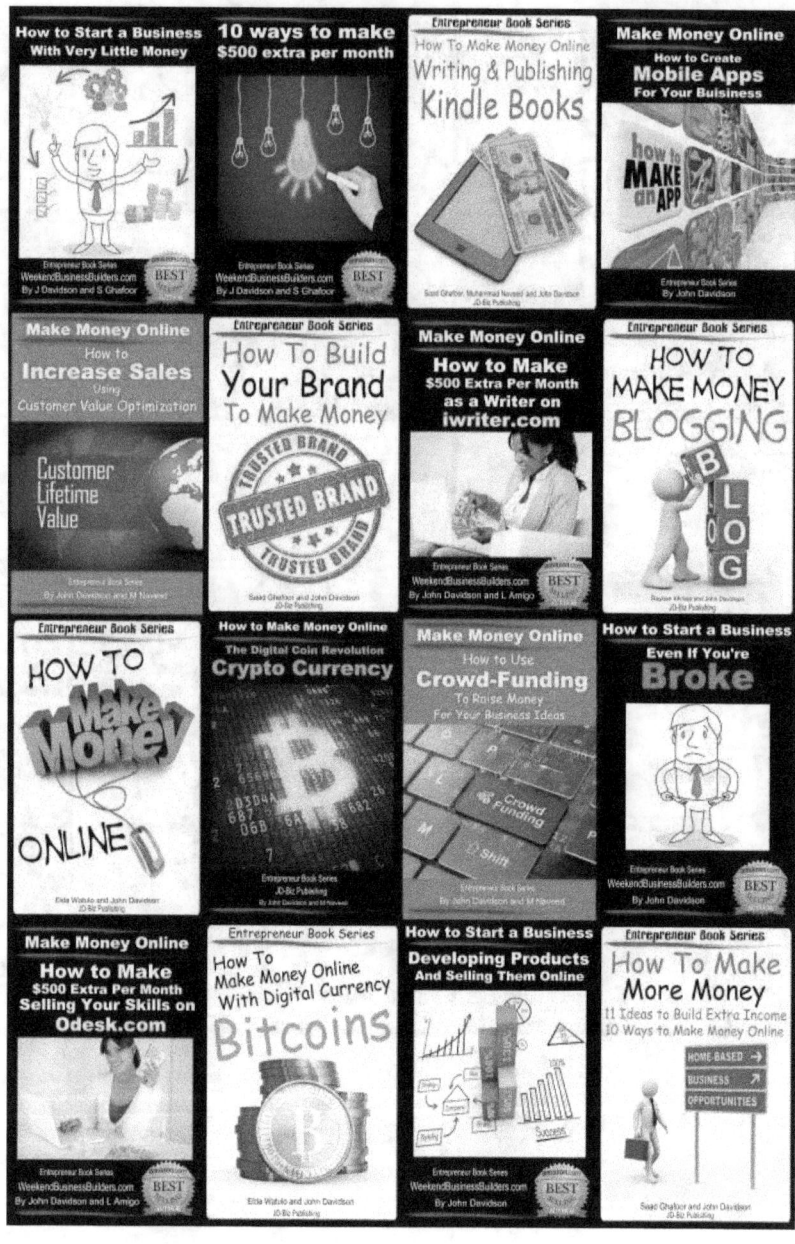

Our books are available at

1. Amazon.com

2. Barnes and Noble

3. Itunes

4. Kobo

5. Smashwords

6. Google Play Books

Download Free Books!

http://MendonCottageBooks.com

Publisher

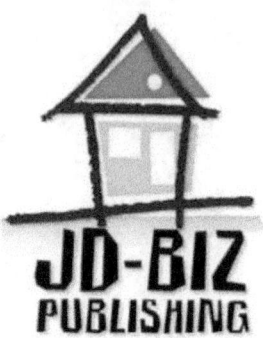

JD-Biz Corp

P O Box 374

Mendon, Utah 84325

http://www.jd-biz.com/

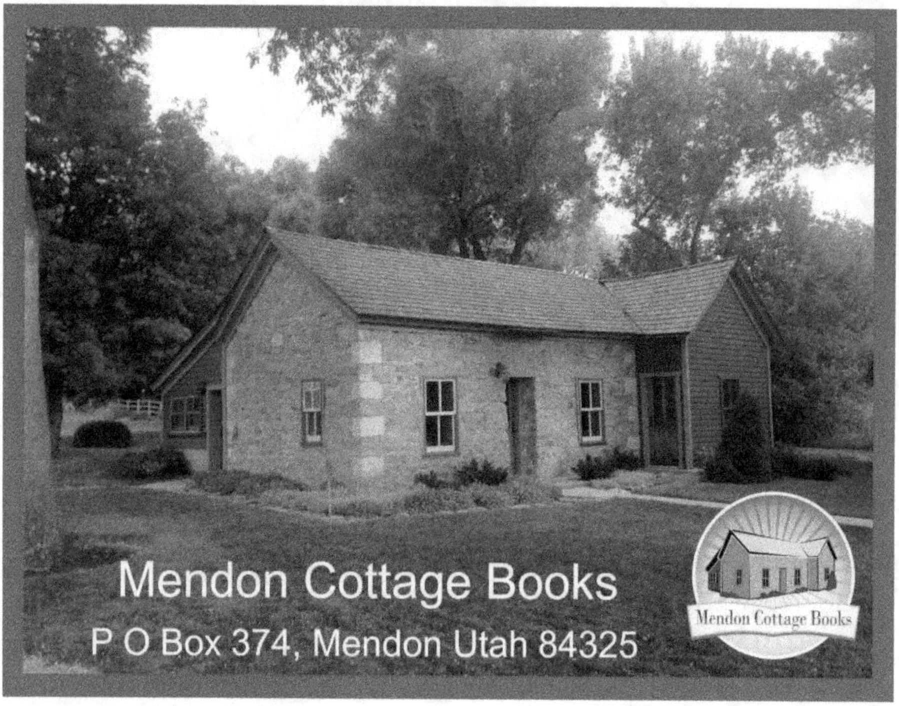

Mendon Cottage Books

P O Box 374, Mendon Utah 84325